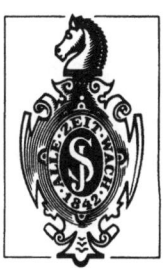

P.P. Abraham L.A. Okoniewski M. Lehman

Cognitive Synthesis Test

With a Foreword by L. Bellak

Springer-Verlag
Berlin Heidelberg New York
London Paris Tokyo

Pamela Pressley Abraham, Psy. D.
Director of Psychological Services
Mapleton Psychiatric Institute, Devereux Foundation
461 Levering Mill, Bala Cynwyd, PA 19004, USA

Lisa Anne Okoniewski, Ph. D.
Clinical Psychologist, Private Practice
4951 McKean Avenue, Philadelphia, PA 19144, USA

Mark Lehman, Ph. D.
Clinical Psychology Intern, Devereux Foundation
625 Wilson Road, Humble, TA 77338, USA

ISBN-13: 978-3-540-17330-4   e-ISBN-13: 978-3-642-71740-6
DOI: 10.1007/978-3-642-71740-6

Library of Congress Cataloging in Publication Data. Main entry under title: Abraham, P. P. (Pamela Pressley), 1951- . Cognitive synthesis test. Bibliography: p.   1. Cognition disorders–Diagnosis. 2. Schizophrenia–Diagnosis. 3. Cognition–Testing. I. Okoniewski, L. A. (Lisa Anne), 1953- . II. Lehman, M. (Mark), 1955- .   III. Title.   [DNLM: 1. Cognition Disorders–diagnosis. 2. Psychological Tests–instrumentation. 3. Schizophrenic Psychology. WM   145   A159c]   RC553.C64A27   1987   616.89'8075 86-31458

© Springer-Verlag Berlin Heidelberg 1987

Typesetting and printing: Druckhaus Beltz, Hemsbach

2119/3140-543210

Foreword

The Cognitive Synthesis Test (CST) started out with a sound clinical observation by its authors: the tolerance of some schizophrenics for incongruencies in thoughts and feelings. The authors then designed pictures which lend themselves to a study of cognitive processes involved in congruent phenomena and of the nature and degree of disruption in goal-directed thinking.

On my first look at the designs and the verbalizations of several patients, I was immediately struck with the richness of the data provided by this test. The pictures present the patient with a task and permit us to study the patient's way of coping, to assess the degree of his/her difficulty in thinking, to examine the nature of the difficulty, and, more generally, to study the problems of integration and synthesis.

Naturally, the patients' stories provide not only formal data but also as a dividend, material useful for their dynamic content. The CST is indeed a brilliantly conceived test with numerous potential applications.

In the long run, quantification should make it possible to use the CST to follow the course of the illness. Also, I think it might be a sensitive instrument for assessing the effect of neuroleptic drugs on cognition. This is a most desirable goal, since we do not know enough about either the constructive effect of these various drugs or the harmful effects which some of them may well have on some patients. Intelligent, observant patients can sometimes report on these effects, but hard data would be preferable. One of my patients, for instance, knows that when he sees the straight lines of tables as curved, it is time for him to take more medication. On the other hand, many patients complain about disturbances of cognition, especially if they get too much neuroleptic medication. Their complaints are not sufficiently heeded by clinicians.

What I have said above already implies that I believe the CST could be a guide for treatment, not only by medication, but also by psychotherapy, specifically by retraining the thought processes, possibly with the help of computers.

In short, I consider the CST a very helpful instrument for the understanding of some problems of schizophrenia and I believe it will be a very useful tool for all clinicians.

Larchmont, NY, February 1987   Leopold Bellak, M.D.

Clinical Professor of Psychiatry
Albert Einstein College of Medicine/
Montefiore Medical Group
Clinical Professor of Psychology
Postdoctoral Program in Psychotherapy
New York University

Table
of Contents

Introduction

Projective tests have been valuable in personality assessment, diagnosis, and treatment by eliciting information about a person's thinking, feelings, fantasies, interests, attitudes, and relationships with others. Picture-story methods such as Murray's Thematic Apperception Test (Murray et al. 1938), The Children's Apperception Test (Bellak and Bellak 1950), Van Lennep's Four-Picture Test (1956), Pickford Projective Pictures (1963), The Object Relations Technique (Phillipson 1956), and Symonds Picture-Story Test (1948) have proven to be successful in revealing underlying personality dynamics.

The Cognitive Synthesis Test (CST) appears to be an innovative and effective technique for evoking verbalizations by means of pictorial material. It offers the opportunity to study fantasy material of psychotic and schizophrenic adolescents, as well as patients in other diagnostic categories.

Development and Rationale

The CST was initially developed to elicit more verbalizations from highly disturbed adolescent patients in an effort to better understand, diagnose, and treat their maladaptive patterns of thoughts, feelings, and actions. Schizophrenic and psychotic patients' attachment to fragmented, seemingly disconnected objects, inanimate objects, and their particular propensity to animate the inanimate world spawned the original idea behind the formulation of the CST. The fact that these patients easily thought in incongruencies, and were often comfortable holding two opposing ideas in their mind, with a minimal need for resolution, further influenced the development of the technique. Thus, the examination of cognitive processes in terms of incongruent linking phenomena and specific disruptions in goal-directed thinking became a focus in the design of the test.

In developing a technique for understanding the adaptive abilities and thought processes of schizophrenic and psychotic patients, it became clear that ego function scales (Bellak et al. 1973), and in particular the synthesis-integration concept, greatly contributed to a meaningful analysis of the material. The synthetic-integrative function of the ego refers to the capacity to assimilate alien elements, mediate between opposing elements, reconcile opposites, find logical connections, and simplify cognitions. The smooth and efficient operation of the synthetic-integrative function is thought to allow for overall economical ego operation by resolving contradictions in thought, feeling, and action (Nunberg 1930). Disruptions in the synthetic function are seen most frequently in children and severely disturbed patients, both of whom have incomplete or weak ego development. However, Nunberg (1930) argued that a failure of synthetic functioning is apparent in all mental symptom formation, and over the years other authors have also linked disturbances in the synthetic ego function with mental illness. Bleuler's (1911) choice of the term "schizophrenia" over "dementia praecox" indicates the importance he placed on integrative operations. The failure to integrate cognitive operations led to a splitting of mental functions, and hence the word "schizophrenia". Similarly, both Klein (1946) and Fairbairn (1952) stress that ego splitting is necessary for the development of psychopathology, particularly with respect to schizoid pathology. Although some degree of ego splitting is found in everyone, the crucial issue is the level at which the splitting occurs. Silverman (1964) posits that a balance between synthesis and splitting is necessary for normal psychological functioning. A prolonged imbalance between these forces can result in psychopathology. Finally, Erickson (1956) defined splitting as closely related to identity diffusion: "In identity diffusion a split of self-images is suggested, a loss of centrality, a sense of dispersion and confusion and a fear of dissolution" (1956, pp. 122–123).

The above discussion clearly emphasizes the significance of the synthetic-integrative functions of the ego, with respect to both personality development and the genesis of psychopathology. It follows that a psychological technique which directly addresses these ego functions, as well as others, would yield productive data. Therefore, the CST was conceptualized as a task which would tap a person's ability to assimilate their thoughts about unrelated images and to express these ideas verbally through story composition.

The choice of stimuli used for the test stemmed from clinical observations, previous research findings, and psychological theories. One of the hallmarks of psychotic disturbances is social withdrawal and an inability to form meaningful attachments with others. This inability to relate interpersonally has its etiology in early psychological development, where problems in object relations are first noted. Many writers (e.g., Mahler 1963, 1968; Bowlby 1969; Burlingham and Freud 1944; Winnicott 1965) have stressed the relationship between deficits in early object relations and subsequent psychopathology. For the psychotic patient, this scenario may be exaggerated to an extreme degree. Searles (1960) notes that these individuals may unconsciously picture themselves as nonhuman, and may then project this picture on the environment. Thus, the psychotic patient perceives others as inhuman, avoiding eye contact, conversation, physical closeness, etc. This avoidance of human contact may be responsible, at least in part, for the brief, unelaborate responses which psychotic patients often give when presented with projective stimuli that incorporate human figures.

Several research efforts support this conclusion. Four studies have addressed the differences in psychotic patients' reactions to human and nonhuman stimuli. Davis and Harrington (1957) examined conceptual discrimination among schizophrenics and normals. They found that schizophrenics were severely disrupted by human stimuli, whereas normals were not. Similarly, Marx (1962) examined the performance of a conceptual task by acute and chronic schizophrenics. The data indicated that human stimuli disrupted the acute schizophrenics more than the chronic schizophrenics. Whiteman (1954) had normals and schizophrenics learn formal concepts (based on physical properties or size relationships) and social concepts (based on interactions among people). Although the schizophrenics' performance was poorer than that of the normals on both tasks, it was significantly worse on tasks involving human concepts. Finally, Brodsky (1961) examined nonpsychotic patients and schizophrenics on conceptual tasks involving human and nonhuman stimuli. The schizophrenics' performance was far worse than that of the nonpsychotic patients in the task involving human stimuli. There was no difference between the groups in the task which employed nonhuman stimuli.

These findings, when viewed in conjunction with clinical observation of psychotic withdrawal and various object relations theories, indicate the need for nonhuman stimuli when assessing seriously disturbed populations. However, a review of available tests (Mitchell 1985) reveals that there are no projective techniques available which use this type of stimulus.

Therefore, with these considerations in mind, the following stimuli were selected for inclusion in the CST:

Card I	Seashell–Watch–Spoon
Card II	Earth–Thermometer–Paperclip
Card III	Leaf–Timer–Arrow
Card IV	Saturn–Hourglass–Electric Socket
Card V	Tornado–Musical Notes–Safety Pin
Card VI	Fire–Glass Clock–Chain
Card VII	Lightning Bolt–Pocket Watch–Wheel
Card VIII	Moon–Ruler–Faucet

Stimulus Choice and Rationale

The objects represented on the eight cards have been divided into three categories: natural elements, objects of time, communication and measurement, and utilitarian items (e.g., tools). The first group are constant forces and elements which belong to the world of nature and which symbolize the universal identification process with natural phenomena. These elements have a significant impact because they respond to their own physical laws independent of human control.

The second category comprises man-made items that have recognizable functions related to time, communication, and measurement. They function to superimpose boundaries on universal dimensions of the world such as time, weight, temperature, thought, and sound. The symbolic components of the objects (numbers, letters, notes) communicate these dimensions concretely according to human need. The form of these items changes over time; however, they are always measuring and communicating permanent dimensions of the world.

The third category is characterized as tools which can be manipulated and utilized for a determined purpose. They have a concrete function toward the accomplishment of a specific result. Goal-directed, logical thought processes are required in order to manipulate these tools successfully.

The purpose of this test is to examine the synthesizing function of thought processes and other ego mechanisms. The objects represented on the cards are not connected by an obvious common denominator, and hence the subject must create an inclusive story which expresses his/her own projections and provides the missing link between the objects. For example, the primary process thinking of the schizophrenic may omit the separateness of the objects through omnipotent, animistic, and narcissistic thinking. These processes undo a clear separation between the objects and forge a common element according to the wishes of the individual. At times, for the psychotic, logic is undone and the wish runs supreme. Boundaries, purpose, and function are subordinated to the dictates of what the schizophrenic wants the objects to do. The wish influences the outcome of the story by curbing the reality value of each object. For example, nature may become a tool, a tool may become communication, and time may bend to the purpose of the story. Thus, while higher functioning persons may attempt to relate between the demands of nature, the reaction in time, and the purpose of the tool, the more regressed person may forego those distinct functions and combine them without logical order or consequence.

Administration

The CST consists of eight cards with three inanimate objects represented on each card. The cards are presented one at a time to an individual in numerical order. The person is told: "I'm going to show you some pictures of objects and I want you to create or make up a story about these objects. I want you to relate the objects in a story." If there are long pauses during the story-telling process, the examiner may repeat the last phrase that was spoken to elicit completion of a sentence or story. Following the story, the examiner then states, "How does your story end; what happens to these three objects?" Responses made during the association portion of the test, as well as any verbal exchange, are recorded verbatim.

The above administration procedures for the CST apply to all the various uses of the cards. These uses include:

1. diagnosis,
2. personality assessment,
3. as a therapeutic tool,
4. as an index of thought organization skills,
5. as a measure for therapeutic improvement, and
6. as a means to gather information in a clinical interview.

References

Bellak L, Bellak SS (1949) Manual of instruction for the children's apperception test. CPS, New York

Bellak L, Hurvich M, Gediman H (1973) Ego functions in schizophrenics, neurotics, and normals. Wiley, New York

Bleuler E (1911) Dementia praecox or the group of schizophrenia. Reprinted: International University, New York, 1950

Bowlby J (1969) Attachment and loss, vol. 1. Basic Books, New York

Brodsky MJ (1961) Interpersonal stimuli as interferences in a sorting task. Dissertation Abstract 22: 2068

Burlingham D, Freud A (1944) Infants without families. Tinling, London

Davis RH, Harrington RW (1957) The effect of stimulus loss on the problem-solving behavior of schizophrenics and normals. Social Psychol 54: 126–128

Erickson E (1956) The problem of ego identity. Psychoanal Ass 4: 56–121

Fairbairn R (1952) The object relations theory of the personality. Basic Books, New York

Klein M (1946) Notes on some schizoid mechanisms. Int J Psychoanal 27: 99–110

Mahler MS (1963) Thoughts about development and individuation. Psychoanal Study Child 18: 307–324

Mahler MS (1968) On human symbiosis and the vicissitudes of individuation. International University Press, New York

Marx A (1962) The effect of interpersonal contact on conceptual task performance of schizophrenics. Doctoral dissertation, University of Oklahoma (unpublished)

Mitchell JV (1985) Ninth mental measurement yearbook. Buros Institute of Mental Measurement, University of Nebraska, Lincoln, Nebraska

Murray HA, Barrett WG, Homburger E, et al. (1938) Explorations in personality. Oxford University Press, New York

Nunberg H (1930) The synthetic function of the ego. In: The practice and theory of psychoanalysis. International University Press, New York, 1960

Phillipson H (1956) The object relations technique (and plates). Tavistock, London

Pickford RW (1963) Pickford projective pictures. Tavistock, London

Searles H (1960) The nonhuman environment. International University Press, New York

Silverman J (1964) The problem of attention in research and theory in schizophrenia. Psychol Rev 71: 352–379

Symonds PM (1948) Symonds picture-story-test. Columbia Bureau of Publications, New York

Whiteman M (1954) The performance of schizophrenics on social concepts. J Abnorm Social Psychol 49: 266–271

Winnicott DW (1965) The maturational process and the facilitating environment. International University Press, New York

Van Lennep DJ (1948) Four-picture test. Lumax, Utrecht

Sample Data for Schizophrenics

Card I: Seashell – Watch – Spoon

R.D.	E.R.	A.N.
Once upon a time there was this seashell lost in the ocean. It was wearing a watch and had a spoon in its mouth eating chocolate. He threw up; he became a butterfly after three wishes from a wizard. *Ending:* He became free with a brand new life.	Once upon a time the seashell was an object of time. The spoon was there to help it. Since it was long the spoon would direct the seashell in time. It would point in a certain direction, the sun would reflect and there appeared a watch. *Ending:* In the end the watch was now a new object of time. It was something the gods of the Greek colony could remember when things were supposed to be.	I see the seashell by the seashore. I see time running out for the seashell because there are not many left. Time will always tell how much time there is to use the spoon to scoop up the sand at the seashore. *Ending:* Let's pretend this is sand. It all ends with a start because there has to be a beginning before there is an end. An end is the beginning.

Card II: Earth – Thermometer – Paperclip

R.D.	E.R.	A.N.
Once upon a time, there was one earth in space. It had a map on it of different parts of the world. Then a thermometer came and made it blow up. The thermometer had hot gases and exploded the earth. Then the thermometer had a paperclip on it and made the paperclip turn to ice. Then the earth went to Heaven and had wings on it and it was flying around Heaven. *Ending:* The earth is flying around Heaven. The ice melted.	The earth where we live next to us the sun reflects, the temperature rises on the thermometer in the far East. They become hotter and hotter, the paperclip melts, the earth is no longer here, people are gone and a new people creates imaginative things around us. *Ending:* The earth is now different. It started with the earth, then the temperature, then the melting of the paperclip.	The planet earth is in space and there is 20 % Fahrenheit for the earth to catch the paperclip. Because time is running at a slow pace and people have to slow down. Then all of a sudden there was a snap, a sound out in space. Then the sounds of thunder crackled and a Norse God Thor appeared and tried to help earth but they didn't believe in him. The earth doesn't believe in good guys 'cause they always finish last. *Ending:* Thor lost his hammer. Now Thor is feeling weak and everyone is making fun of him. The earth started to go haywire and the earth was safe because Spiderman came and found Thor's hammer. Spiderman and Thor saved the earth!

Card III: Leaf – Timer – Arrow

R.D.	E.R.	A.N.
Once upon a time, there was this precious leaf. It had an arrow on it — no, an arrow is pointing toward it. The leaf was running and the timer was testing him to see how fast the leaf could go in 1 minute. The arrow was running out of gas — it was following the leaf! *Ending:* It was the 50-yard dash! They all collapse!	The timer, the leaf, what a relief! Now the arrow is pointing the way; it hates to see us so far away. Now the pain is going away. I wish he (the arrow) wouldn't be so angry; I tried to explain things are rough. I love the leaf like a buff. The leaf loves me, too, 'cause after all I am the time. *Ending:* So, eventually the arrow understood that me and the leaf do not hate him – we only needed time away.	The arrow is pointing toward the time that is running out for the leaf because all things come to an end in time. *Ending:* The arrow is pointing sideways and the leaf is pointing upward. This middle of the leaf is important for the timer. That's where the timer gets its energy.

Card IV: Saturn – Hourglass – Electric Socket

R.D.	E.R.	A.N.
Once upon a time, there was this hourglass underwater and it was magic. Then the hourglass turned the light on underwater and I saw Saturn. The hourglass sat on Saturn and ate a sandwich. The light switch went "peek-a-boo I see you!" *Ending:* They all live happily ever after underwater in the ocean.	I'm not on Saturn. I wish I could leave. The earth seems so far it looks to be like an hourglass of time. If I can leave through the hourglass and through an electrical socket, I could be home like it used to be in 2 flat seconds. *Ending:* I finally left through the hourglass and electrical socket. I passed through it — I saw the people I used to be — now I'm gone and am very happy I shall never return.	One of Saturn's rings is falling apart and it's being timed by the hourglass. One of Saturn's moons crashed into it. The electric plug is connected to the hourglass because Saturn came out of the electric plug and so did the hourglass. *Ending:* Planet exploded because there is something missing because there might be life on Saturn.

Card V: Tornado – Musical Notes – Safety Pin

R.D.	E.R.	A.N.
Once upon a time there came a big tornado with a smile on its face saying notes to itself. It's saying my favorite things — the tornado found a safety pin on the ground and it wished for a candy bar. Then it went away to Heaven and celebrated Thanksgiving. *Ending:* It sang Christmas songs. The tornado vanished. The notes were walking toward the shore to go swimming.	The notes sends out a lovely tune but the tune vibrates to a safety pin. But only the pin knows that the music notes are humming a tune to destruction. Once the pin vibrates, it sends it all over the world — It hits the wrong cloud in the world and forms a tornado. The tornado now destroys the musical notes and the safety pin. *Ending:* The tornado discovered that the safety pin and the notes were looking for trouble. But now the tornado has ceased and the destruction of the world has also ceased.	The twister is coming toward the musical notes and it's saying we have to clip on to something because time is running out. We need something to hold onto. The twister (this is God's love). God is saying to the twister you got to hang onto the safety pin or time will run out and there will be nothing to hang onto. *Ending:* The twister made it through all the space storms. The twister got to the musical notes and they are held into the twister but the safety pin is left in space. But God reached out and grabbed everything and brought it back to wherever God lives. He freed the twister — if you love something you set it free. If you think you can, you can. It all comes naturally.

Card VI: Fire – Glass Clock – Chain

R.D.	E.R.	A.N.
Once upon a time there was this clock. It tick-tocked and said "Oh, heck, how did I become a clock." Then fire burned it up – then the fire ate up the chain. Then the fire said "Oh boy, what a wonderful meal!" *Ending:* They all vanish into fire dust. The chain said "Zipidy-do-dah — my oh my, what a wonderful day."	The clock says the time of 5:00 p.m. It now told the chain to pull against the world's enemy. The enemy was the fire. The fire shall destroy once the clock gets 6:00. The fire is now spreading through tons of woods and tons of houses. The chain pulls against the fire and out the fire goes because it's time now at 6:00. *Ending:* You shall never see the fire again until the clock hits 5:00 again.	The clock stands for all the time left in the world. The chain was left by one of the Devil's friends. One of the Devil's exfriends turned into one of God's enemies. The fire is the Devil's only friend. He hurt God — that's why God is always upset because God's children suffer all the time. They are hurrying, tired, overworked and they find it hard to care about each other because of confidence. *Ending:* The fire is ready to burn out. The chains are shackles broken by time. God and the Devil had a fight. The Devil put a trick on God and yanked him out of Heaven.

Card VII: Lightning Bolt – Pocket Watch – Wheel

R.D.	E.R.	A.N.
Once upon a time there was this precious light bulb. It carried a watch that fits in its pocket. Then it met a wheel running down the street. Then it said "Hi" to the pocket watch. The wheel asked the light bulb to dance with him then the pocket watch timed them on the 50-yard dash and off they went. *Ending:* The light bulb, watch and wheel won a gold medal in the 50-yard dash. The light bulb ran the fastest — in 58 seconds.	The time now is 2:00 p.m. There was a watch for a storm and everything they said (the people) would be destroyed. It's all in God's power to prevent this so now the lightning has begun. It has hit the wheel. The wheel served the turning pin for gas and oil. *Ending:* Lightning stopped. The clock is turned and the wheel has served its purpose and the people are all safe again, thanks to God.	All of a sudden on a nice quiet day in Vermont — all of a sudden there was a storm and a wheel was rolling down the hill and an old man had a pocket watch in his shirt. There was a small child at the top of the hill and the old man was at the bottom of the hill. The child got upset about the storm — The lightning bolt struck between the child and the old man. *Ending:* There was a bird in the sky and landed on the old man's hand. The child said how did you do that — the old man pulled out his watch and said — I have to go.

Card VIII: Moon – Ruler – Faucet

R.D.	E.R.	A.N.
Once upon a time, there was this faucet and out of it came pink water and then it turned yellow. And there was this little moon that spun around in circles — then came a ruler and sat on the moon. The moon said "Get the heck off me — will you?" The ruler sits back and the moon comes up to it and says, "Hi, sweetheart, how are you?" The faucet says "Turn me on — turn me off" to the moon and ruler. *Ending:* The moon and the ruler says "Let's hit the road Jack!" The faucet changed into a butterfly; it was green.	There was a man which was the ruler from the moon. He liked to measure things. One time his measuring turned to destruction. He walked around till he came to a faucet. The faucet was asleep and the moon was awake and so was the ruler. But anyway, he began measuring the faucet and the faucet woke up and down tumbled the ruler. The faucet turned on and the ruler drowned but the moon sat in the sky and laughed. *Ending:* So the moon got its serve, payback, or what he deserved — He always liked light so the sun decided to make him be the dark side of the moon.	The ruler measures how much time in space there really was. The moon will be like that tonight. The rain is dripping out of the faucet and the ruler is measuring it and the moon is the source of the water. *Ending:* The water keeps going on and on.

Sample Data for Other Diagnostic Categories

Card I: Seashell – Watch – Spoon

Bipolar disorder (manic/despressive)	Depressed suicidal	Borderline personality
R.O.	M.C.	S.P.
This girl went to the beach and she was wearing her favorite watch on her wrist. She was walking along the edge of water and her wristwatch fell off her arm and she reached down, got her watch and found a silver spoon. She took it to a pawn shop and took it to a store and bought some seashells. Then she went down the block and bought a keg of beer and three Shermans (three joints of PCP). Then she went home and smoked them. Then she took her watch off and took it to a pawn shop and got money and bought more drugs and smoked them and got high and then she died. *Ending:* She died.	A ship sunk and that's the stuff floating down on the bottom of the ocean. The ship got torpedoed. It's been lying on the bottom for 40 years. It's gotten kinda rusty. *Ending:* It has no end. It lies there on the bottom. They just sit there and rust.	Someone was walking along the beach with a metal detector and he found a really huge seashell. He put it in his bag of treasures and went along and it started beeping and he dug in the sand with his hand and found a spoon. Then he started digging with the spoon and found a watch. *Ending:* He takes them home and puts the seashell in a fish tank. The spoon is corroded so he throws it away. He takes the watch to be fixed by his friend, the jeweler, and he wears it forever. So, now he can tell what time it is.

Card II: Earth – Thermometer – Paperclip

Bipolar disorder (manic/despressive)	Depressed suicidal	Borderline personality
R.O.	M.C.	S.P.
There was a scientist and he studied the earth and one day the temperature went way up to 120° and it was so hot. We were all drinking Pepsi! A scientist figured out a way to save us and make the world a normal temperature with a paperclip. Then his paperclip idea fucked up and we all died. *Ending:* He made it cold instead of hot and we all died.	It shows how man's progress is. It's got devices to measure temperature, a device to hold paper together and we can even see what our earth looks like. They (the objects) become more advanced by technology. *Ending:* They become more refined. They are all dug up by archeologists and they think how primitive we are. Or they will find them in an antique shop some day. Thermometers will be around a long time. Nobody will be precise about temperature. They don't want to be — they don't care.	One day we got in a war with the Russians. They made a huge warhead out of a paperclip 50 stories high. They bombed the USA with it. USA retaliated by bombing them. The earth's core just split half open. The guys from outer space came and landed on one of the halves of the earth. The thermometer was their spaceship and they found out that the earth was 10000°. They were radiation monsters which means they live and thrive on radiation and they took all the people still alive and shipped them off to their planet where there is no radiation and let them live there. *Ending:* They took over the earth and the earth people took over their planet.

Card III: Leaf – Timer – Arrow

Bipolar disorder (manic/despressive)	Depressed suicidal	Borderline personality
R.O.	M.C.	S.P.
There was this huge gigantic leaf and this girl and guy got on it and they were screwing. Then they were in the middle of the woods and a kitchen time clock went off and they freaked out and this big arrow was sticking in the ground and said to go left. Then there was this big, big, big, big, etc. huge restaurant that looked just like a time clock and they went in and ate leaves; of course only maple and cherry leaves. Then there was a big arrow that told them which way to get out. *Ending:* She umm… went out there and threw up because of the leaves. They got on the big leaf and screwed some more.	This is the fall and the timer. Well, somebody is cooking something, an apple pie. The arrow is pointing in the direction of the food. *Ending:* Reminds me of visiting my grandmother in Northern Pennsylvania. The leaves had fallen off the trees and the arrow points where I can get my eats. Time means death. The longer you live the closer you get to death.	There was this family and they had a pet leaf. They lived on a one-way street. The leaf got sick. The leaf hospital was at the other end of the street. They had to go the wrong way on the one-way street to get to the hospital. The father got half way up the street and a policeman stopped him and gave him a ticket for going the wrong way on a one-way street. He had 5 min to get to the hospital and had to take all these detours to get there. (The leaf got sick and was going to die in 5 min.) He kept looking at the timer which kept saying 5 min. *Ending:* He keeps driving and he finally gets to the hospital. The timer said 5 min — little did he know the battery was dead, and so was the leaf.

Card IV: Saturn – Hourglass – Electric Socket

Bipolar disorder (manic/despressive)	Depressed suicidal	Borderline personality
R.O.	M.C.	S.P.
There's a rocket and it is timed by an hourglass and has 30 sec. to get to Saturn. The rocket goes off and gets there in 30 sec. They stop at the little lines that go around Saturn to get gas, hamburgers and french fries, and Star Bursts. Then they go to Saturn and one of the ladies on the rocket has to wash and blow dry her hair cause it was dirty and then she plugged it into the wall. She had been wet cause one of the men on the way into Saturn squeezed all the oil out of the hamburger. It got all over her. When she plugged it in her hair stood up because the cord dropped on her wet arm. *Ending:* She went back out into the rocket, got in and hit the man that did that to her.	The hourglass symbolized the passage of time that it takes Saturn about 20–30 years to go around the sun. We've invented electricity and we've invented machines to measure time. We've gone a long way and are waiting to go to Saturn to make things happen. *Ending:* It ends with monotony — just waiting.	Many moons ago these funny-shaped objects came from the sky and landed on the earth in the country of Egypt and told the Egyptians the secret of electricity, pyramids and time. They taught the more intelligent Egyptians mathematical equations for making the first electric hourglass. *Ending:* So the Egyptians used their mathematical equations and theory of time to come up with the first electric clock to be plugged into the first electric wall socket.

Card V: Tornado – Musical Notes – Safety Pin

Bipolar disorder (manic/despressive)	Depressed suicidal	Borderline personality
R.O.	M.C.	S.P.
Once upon a time, there was this girl walking along singing a song! Oh! then she reached down and took the safety pin out of her skirt and all of a sudden she turned around and a big tornado was chasing her. She hit the deck and the tornado went over her and swept the safety pin out of her hand. As the tornado went round and round (Oh, That's fun). The safety pin got bigger and bigger and bigger. *Ending:* The tornado started to disintegrate and the safety pin started chasing her back home and the safety pin fell down and the dog chewed it up! Her grandmother helped her fight the safety pin!	The tornado comes while somebody's playing music. The safety pin is just laying on the ground after the tornado hit. *Ending:* Nobody knows what happened to the guy playing music. Nobody cares about the safety pin.	This kid had a trumpet and he was the world's best trumpet player — world renown. He picked up his trumpet and blew it as hard as he could and no music would come out. So he hooked it up to his father's air compressor to get some sound out of it. He got so frustrated that he turned the power beyond maximum power. A huge gust of wind came out and turned into a tornado. It ripped the town in half except for his house of course. *Ending:* Investigators came to find out why his house was not destroyed and to find out how it started. He said he put the air compressor to his trumpet and a tornado came out. The experts said aerodynamically it's impossible to start a tornado like that and were amazed and wanted to use it as a weapon. When they looked into the trumpet there was a safety pin and that's what caused the special aerodynamic effects.

Card VI: Fire – Glass Clock – Chain

Bipolar disorder (manic/despressive)	Depressed suicidal	Borderline personality
R.O.	M.C.	S.P.
At 8:00, no, at 10:00 Laura, Jill, Bryan and Mike went out in the woods to build a campfire. Then, as they were sitting around in the darkness they heard chains rattling and footsteps in the woods. They got all scared; they ran out to the car and got in and locked the doors. They started making out. This girl got pregnant and they went home. *Ending:* She has an abortion and her mom yells at her. Do you love me?	Somebody's chained to a wall and the house is on fire. The clock shows how much time is left. It's just time left. He's counting the minutes till the fire gets him. *Ending:* Thats the end — he's counting the minutes.	There was three inmates at a State Prison. They all decided they would escape one night. And they got out of the prison and the sirens went on and also the searchlights. Then all of a sudden the electricity went off. So the guards set the field on fire so they could see the inmates. So they started shooting and killed two of them and one got out with a bullet in his back. He went to a different country to have an operation and the country was known for a glass clock with a gold pendulum. *Ending:* He stole the clock. Sold the gold pendulum in another country and then went back and got the operation. He lived happily ever after except that his hands were chained together.

Card VII: Lightning Bolt – Pocket Watch – Wheel

Bipolar disorder (manic/despressive)	Depressed suicidal	Borderline personality
R.O.	M.C.	S.P.
This little nerdy boy — he took a wagon wheel and went out one night with his pocket watch and was waiting for the big storm. He could tell the storm was coming by the air. He was waiting and waiting for the storm. It thundered and lightninged and it hit him on the head and then it knocked him on his butt! When he woke up he took a joint out and started smoking it and he got high! *Ending:* He went home and went to sleep — (she began to sing) Roll, roll, roll your joint, pass it down the line, take a toke, hold your smoke, blow your fuckin' mind!!! I love rhymes, do you?	It's in a field and a wagon wheel is laying around. Somebody's looking at their watch and a storm is -coming. They go home for dinner. *Ending:* He goes home for dinner.	There was this stagecoach bringing very important persons (VIPs) to Texas. Lightning hit the front wheel and knocked the wheel off. *Ending:* So the driver took his watch and attached it to the axle in place of the wheel. They then went merrily on their way. It soon became the size of a pocket watch and was the first mobile watch.

Card VIII: Moon – Ruler – Faucet

Bipolar disorder (manic/despressive)	Depressed suicidal	Borderline personality
R.O.	M.C.	S.P.
Once there was this scientist and he got his ruler and he went outside at night and he measured the moon and got carried away and measured everything in sight! He went back inside his house and he got a cup and put ice in it and put water in it. He even measured the ice cube but it kept melting! He went back outside and he measured some more and drank all the water up. *Ending:* He threw the cup down and went inside and jerked off and went to bed.	It's in a school building at night and all that's left is a dripping faucet and ruler. It's at night and the moon is shining down on it. Nobody is there. It is all quiet. *Ending:* Dawn comes.	This guy tried to measure the moon while running water on his ruler because he had dry skin. *Ending:* He flooded the moon and it became too heavy to stay in the earth's atmosphere because it was too destructive. A space shuttle went up and attached two rocket boosters and sent it twirling off into outer space.

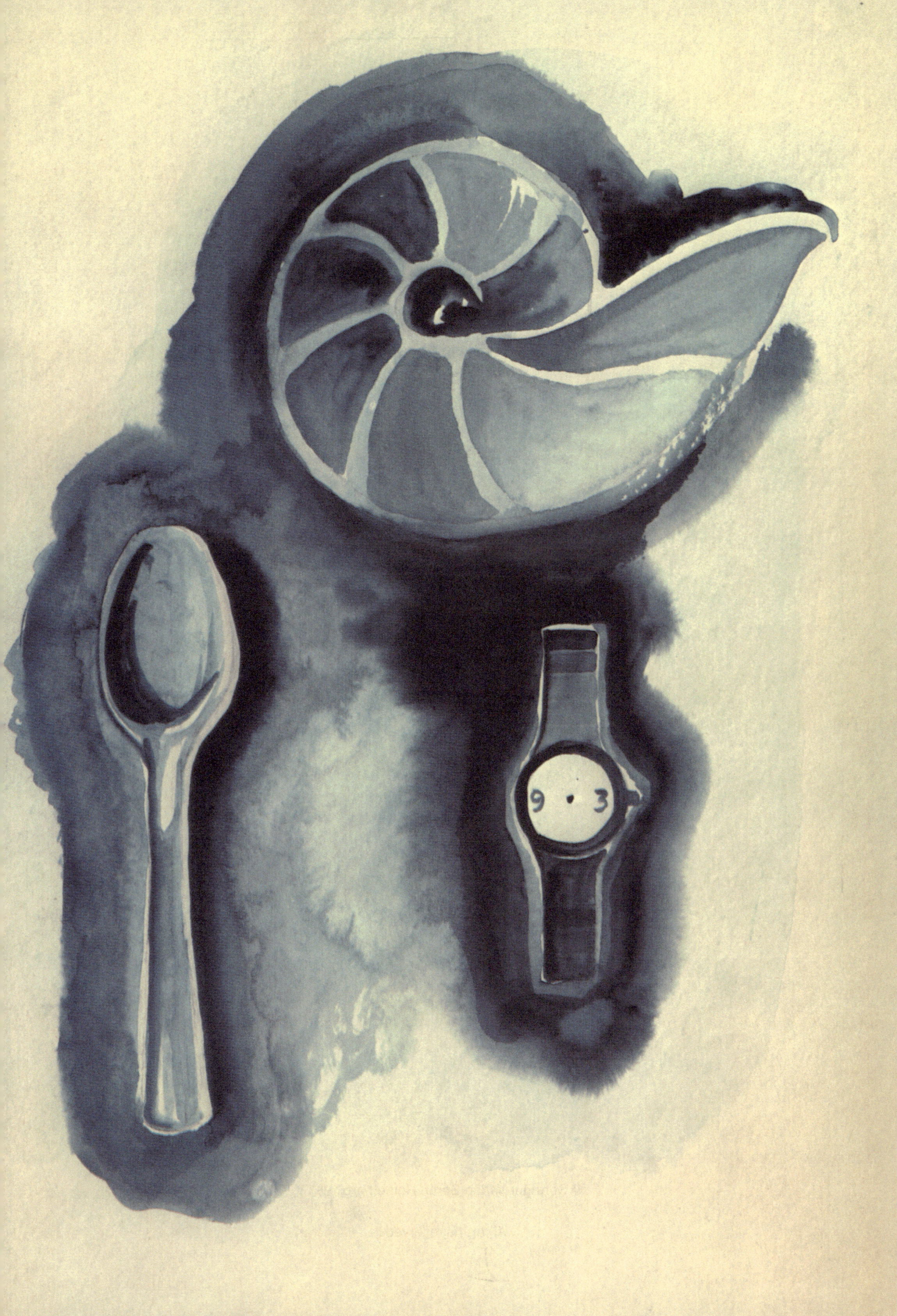

Card I Seashell – Watch – Spoon

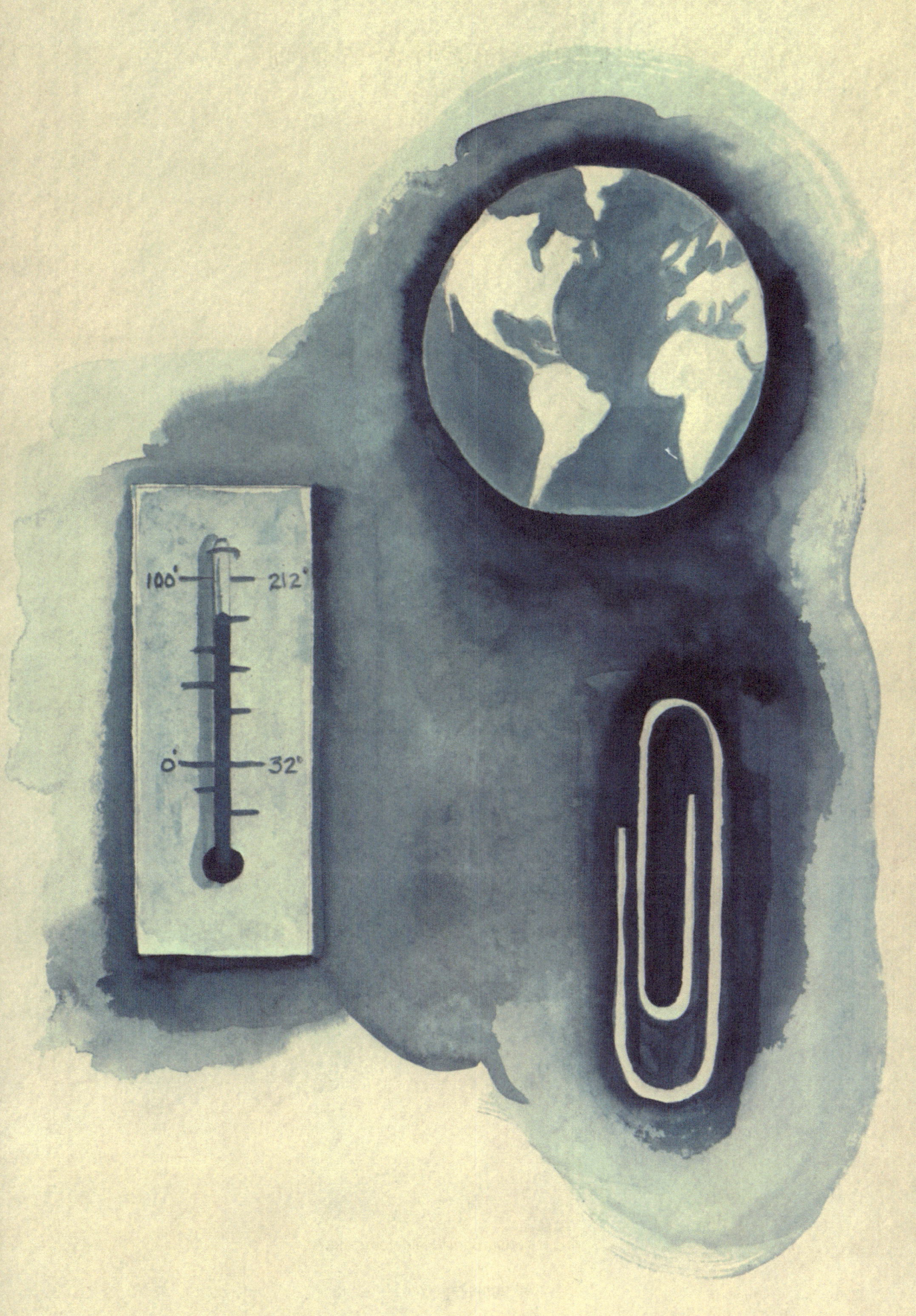

Card II Earth – Thermometer – Paperclip

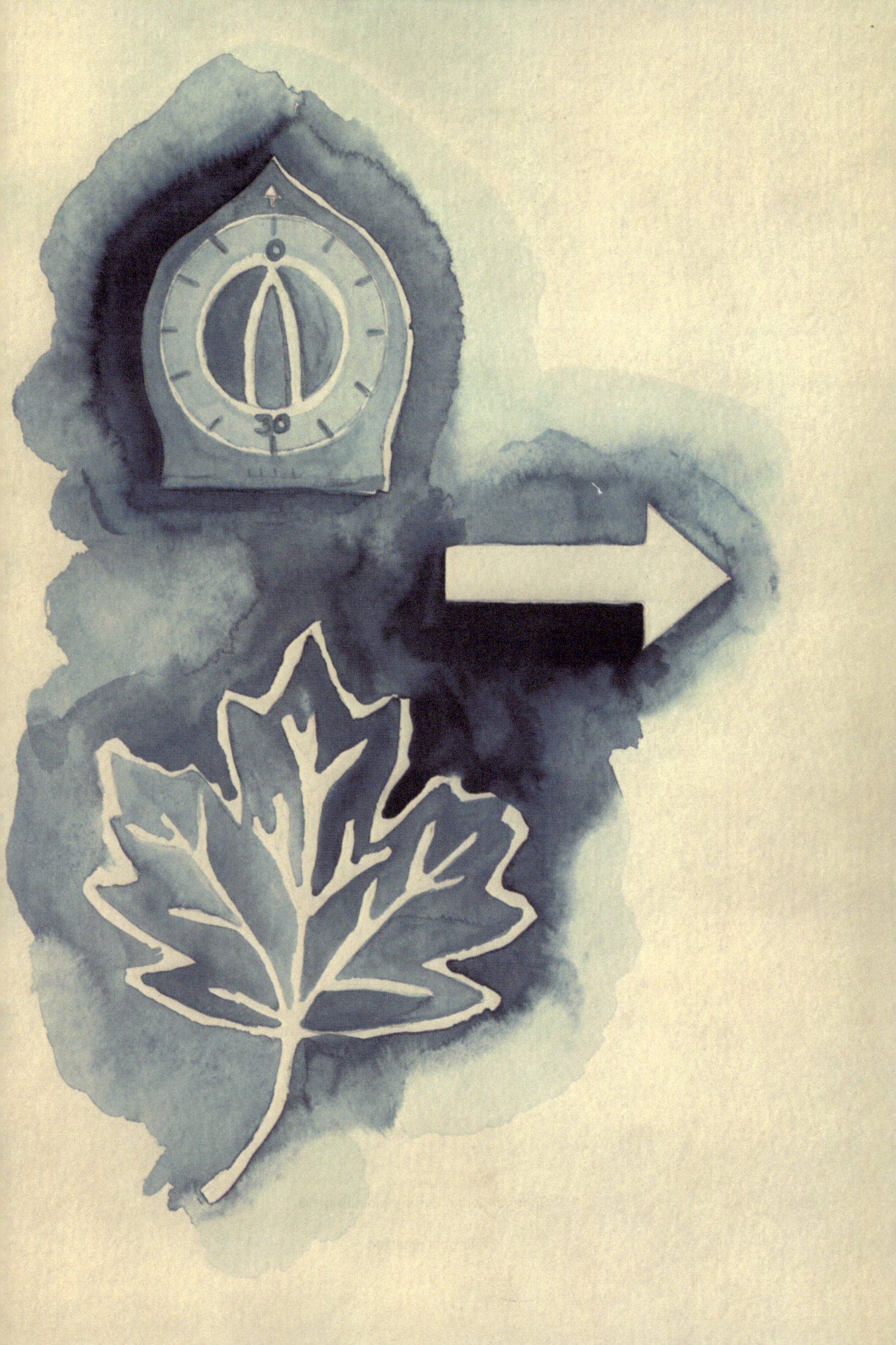

Card III Leaf – Timer – Arrow

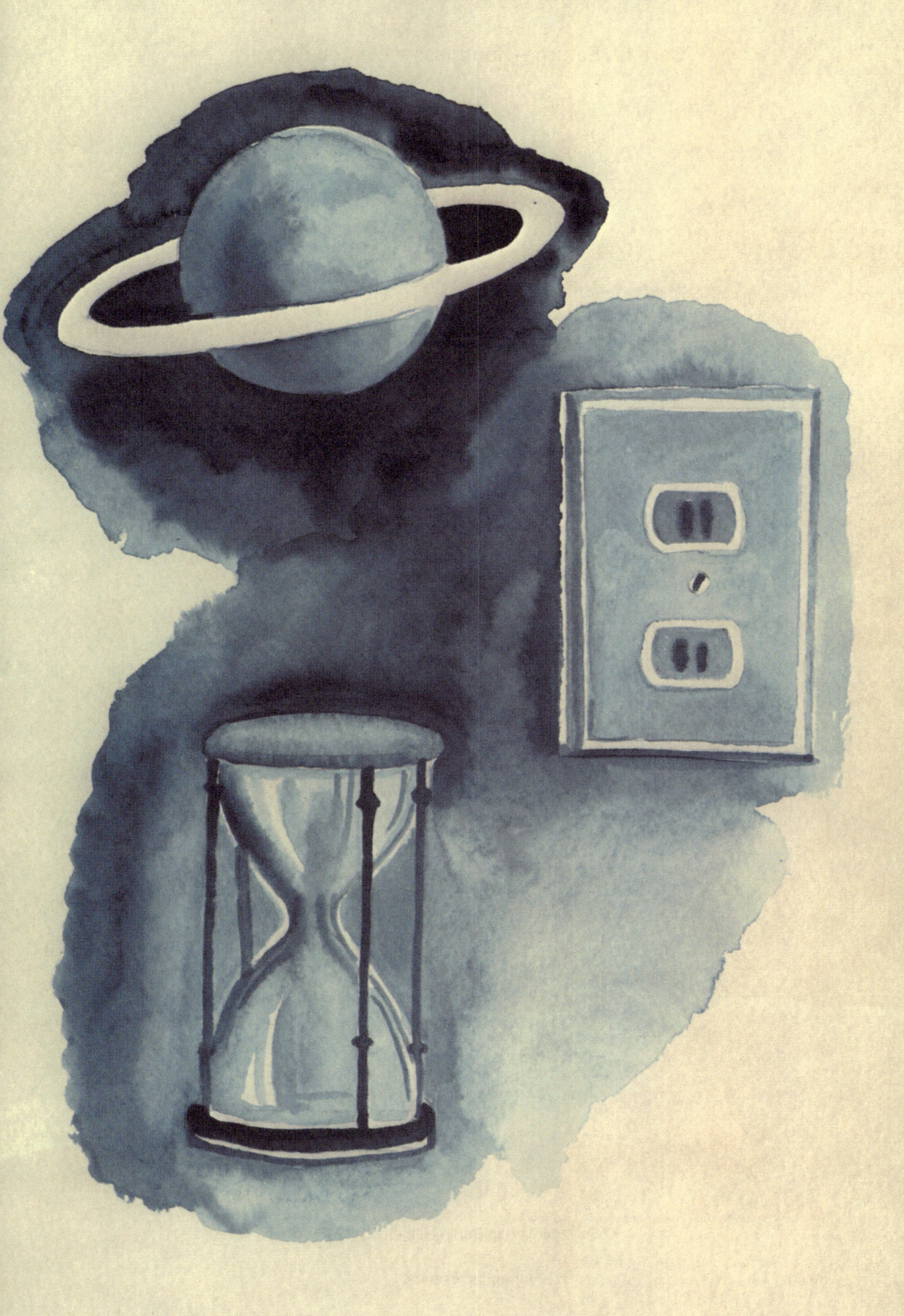

Card IV Saturn – Hourglass – Electric Socket

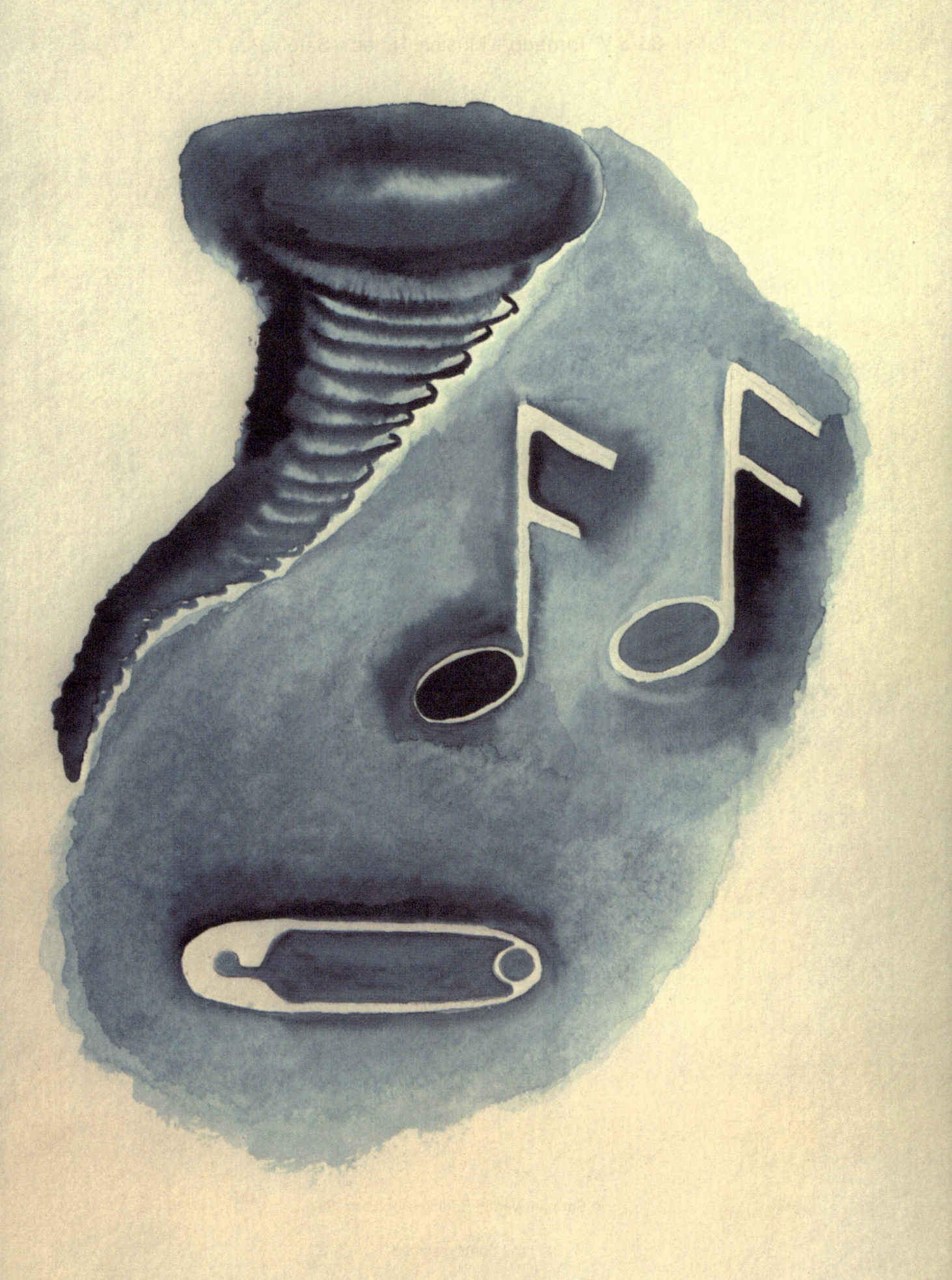

Card V Tornado – Musical Notes – Safety Pin

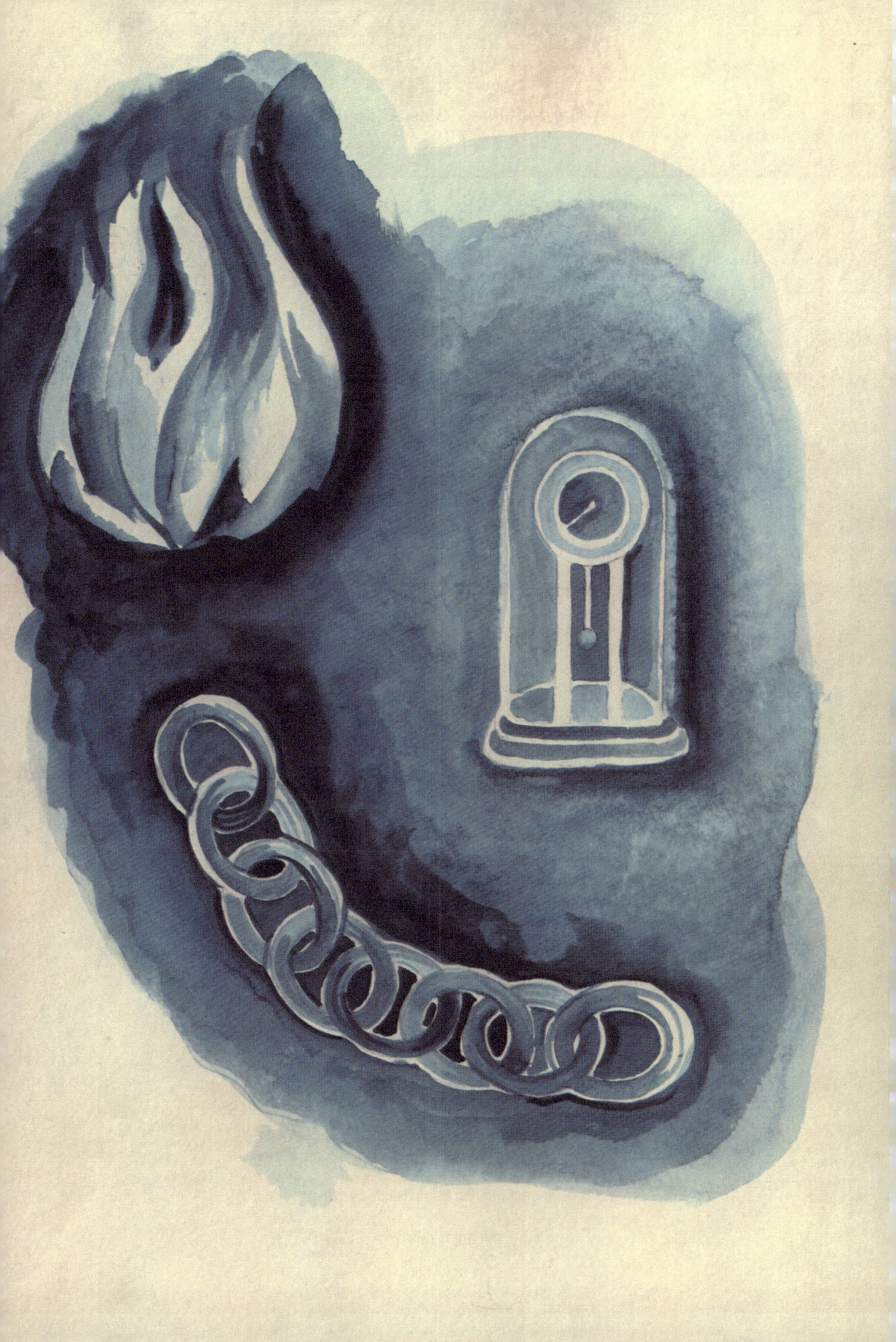

Card VI Fire – Glass Clock – Chain

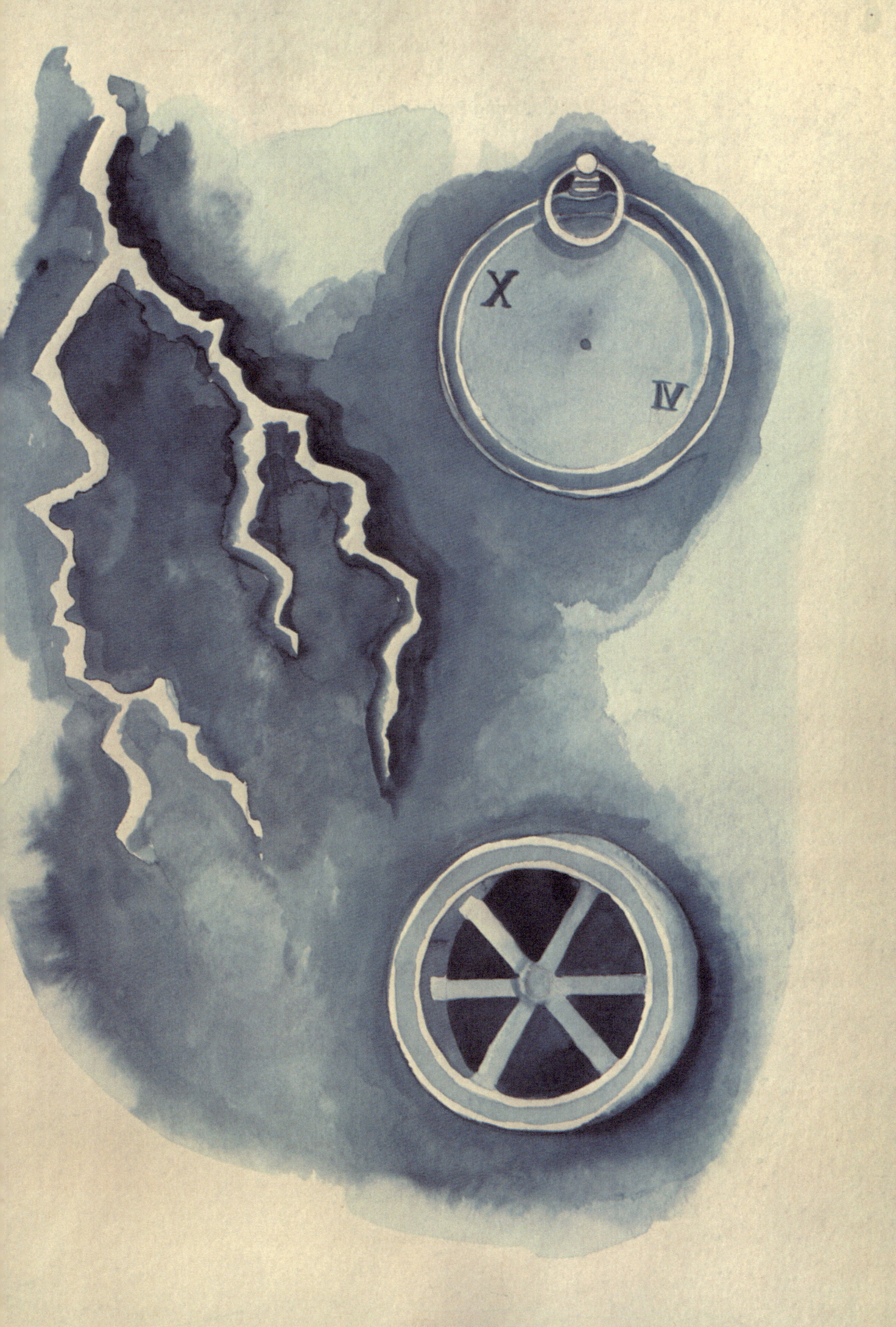

Card VII Lightning Bolt – Pocket Watch – Wheel

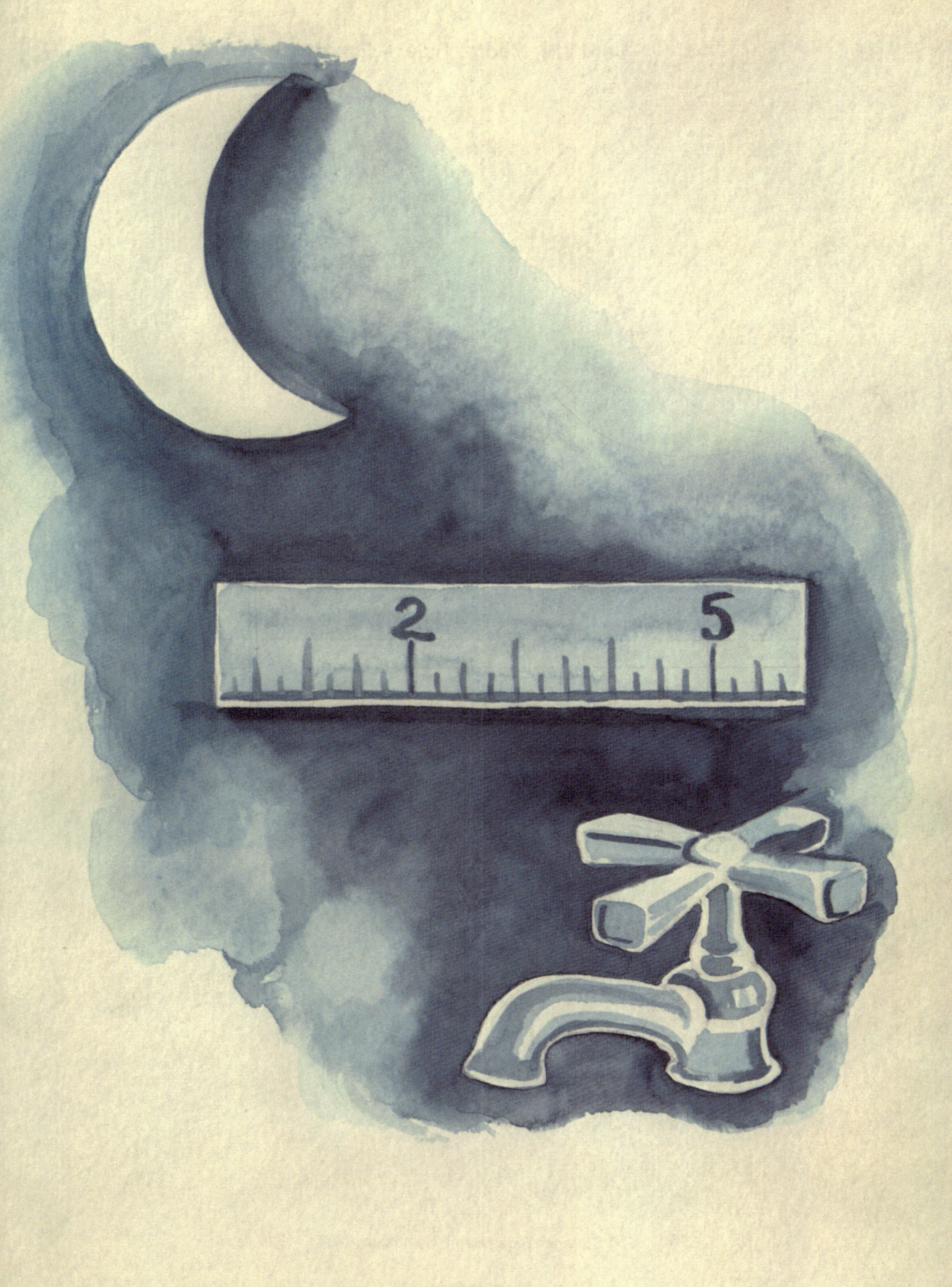

Card VIII Moon – Ruler – Faucet